What Others a

Dancing Upon Barren Land is a necessary tool for anyone struggling with baby hunger. Through her own experience, author Lesli Westfall gives the reader the words that grief has stolen.**—Beth Forbus, Sarah's Laughter, Christian Support for Infertility & Child Loss**

Dancing Upon Barren Land ~ Prayer, Scripture Reflections and Hope for Infertility is a valuable resource for any woman feeling misunderstood, overlooked, and alone and is a guide to experiencing comfort, solace, and hope during a time of infertility.**—Dr. Paul Osteen, Associate Pastor, Lakewood Church, Houston, Texas**

Lesli is funny, anointed, and an excellent steward of the Word of God.**—Rhonda Nwosu, Sparkles of Life, Inc., Educating and Empowering Couples through Infertility and Delayed Parenting**

Now, I have a deeper understanding of what women are facing and I believe it will equip me better in ministering to those struggling. For the one going through infertility, this book is an invitation from her Maker to "dance" together on this journey and is a path of hope and instruction too.**—Jana Lackey, Co-Founder, Love Botswana Outreach Mission, Maun, Botswana, Africa**

I believe Lesli has a heart to encourage women struggling with infertility, as well as educate family and friends on how best to support their loved ones. Through the pages of *Dancing Upon Barren Land* and the online ministry, it is my prayer for Lesli and all who discover this source that fruitfulness will abound. **—Nerida Walker, New Life Ministries –Bringing Life to Barrenness, Sydney, Australia**

Through the collection of prayers and scripture reflections in this book, the reader will experience peace, balance in his or her relationships, and encouragement to believe in the goodness of God and His power in impossible situations.—**Pastor Jackie Garner, Director of Women's Ministry, Lakewood Church**

Dancing Upon Barren Land is a vital, life changing book I - recommend to every couple struggling with infertility. Lesli so eloquently depicts Jesus' love for all, calling the reader up and out of the struggle to an authentic relationship with Jesus, pointing them to hope in Jesus and God's Word. Through her authenticity and relationship with the Lord, Lesli gives every couple hope that they too can dance upon barren land!—**Adana Wilson, Associate Pastor of Adult Ministries, Gateway Church, Frisco, Texas**

Lesli has a mother's heart for women struggling with infertility. Her love for the Lord and tenacious faith were never more evident when she received news that a fertility treatment did not work. We have watched her walk in faith and she has much to say to women who are struggling with infertility and those who aren't as well, for her years of study and life experience have paid dividends of great wisdom. *Dancing Upon Barren Land* is proof of this wisdom offering a beacon of hope and a tower of strength for those walking alongside her. We are privileged to call her friend.—**The Peeps, Lesli's friends: Becki Guillory, JoAnn Heath, Andrea Jones, Renee Reagan, Heather Volentine**

DANCING UPON BARREN LAND

Dancing Upon Barren Land

~

Prayer, Scripture Reflections, and Hope
for
Infertility

by
Lesli A. Westfall

Dancing Upon Barren Land
P.O. Box 1054
Pearland, Texas 77588

@copyright Lesli A. Westfall 2013

Printed in the U.S.A.

Dancing Upon Barren Land
P.O. Box 1054
Pearland, Texas 77588

Book development: Karen Porter, kae Creative Solutions, kaeporter@gmail.com

Unless otherwise marked, Scripture quotations are taken from the Holy Bible, New International Version®, NIV®. Copyright © 1973, 1978, 1984, 2011 by Biblica, Inc.™ Used by permission of Zondervan. All rights reserved worldwide. www.zondervan.com The "NIV" and "New International Version" are trademarks registered in the United States Patent and Trademark Office by Biblica, Inc.™
Scripture quotations marked AMP are taken from the New American Standard Bible®, Copyright © 1960, 1962, 1963, 1968, 1971, 1972, 1973, 1975, 1977, 1995 by The Lockman Foundation. Used by permission. (www.Lockman.org)
Scripture quotations marked NASB are taken from the New American Standard Bible®, Copyright © 1960, 1962, 1963, 1968, 1971, 1972, 1973, 1975, 1977, 1995 by The Lockman Foundation. Used by permission. (www.Lockman.org)
Scripture quotations marked "KJV" are taken from the Holy Bible, King James Version, Cambridge, 1769.
Scripture quotations market THE MESSAGE are taken from THE MESSAGE, copyright© by Eugene H. Person 1993, 1994, 1995, 1996, 2000, 2001, 2002. Used by permission of NavPress Publishing Group.

This book is dedicated
to the Women of
HOPE ~ Hearts of Promise and Expectation©
Christian Infertility Support Group
at
Lakewood Church, Houston, Texas

Table of Contents

Foreword

I have known the pain and heartache of eight years of infertility, surgeries, and all the marvelous medical treatments available to women today. As a mother, I have also experienced God's wonderful provision as He blessed my husband and me with three children through the miracle of adoption. God promises in Psalm 113:9 *to settle the barren woman in her home as a happy mother of children.* Today I can truly say God made me a happy mother of 14-year-old twin girls and an 11-year-old son.

During those eight years of infertility, I held on to God's Word with my life when every circumstance seemed hopeless. I relished every hope-filled word of encouragement from family and friends. How I wish I'd had this amazing book, *Dancing Upon Barren Land* by my friend, Lesli Westfall. There were times I wanted to feel sorry for myself, but God's Word always strengthened me and sustained me. When I felt like my situation was impossible, I learned to dance upon my barren ground and declare: "I am a happy mother of children."

I have known Lesli many years, as she has been a member of Lakewood Church and Director of our HOPE ~ Hearts of Promise and Expectation© infertility support group. After years of experience, she has beautifully written a resource that will empower you to be filled with hope and God's Word. Lesli's book will show you how to pray and allow God to turn your sorrow into joy and your mourning into dancing, for with Him all things are possible. I know you will be blessed, spiritually strengthened, and encouraged as you read this powerful tool, *Dancing Upon Barren Land*. I encourage you to keep it close by your side and allow it to be a manual you can rely on every day.

God bless you, sustain you, and give you the desires of your heart.

Lisa Osteen Comes
Author, *You Are Made For More!*

Introduction

I'm sure there is a reason you chose this book, either for yourself or for someone you know. I could guess it wasn't the creative title or the beautiful book cover; it's because you saw the word "infertility."

When we deal with infertility, we can stand on the edge of life like a sad wallflower who is never asked to dance, or we can step onto the dance floor, hear the music, and dance upon barren land.

"Ouch." Comparing infertility to dancing? Sometimes our toes get stepped on and it hurts.

I feel for you. Whether you, your spouse, beloved family member, or friend is struggling with infertility, I empathize with you. In this book, I honestly express my heart about what I have been through and am still going through. I thought I could choreograph the dance steps, but I've realized the ordered steps of this barren road have not been a dance of my own choosing; instead, it has been a dance I didn't want to learn. And the journey is one of misunderstanding, too, especially because I am a born-again Christian. I know God loves me, yet I still find myself from time to time asking the question, "Why, God? Why?"

I wish I had the answers to all your questions, but I don't. Even though I don't understand the why, I do know the Who. The Who is God, the lead partner of the dance.

When we stumble, God is the One who knows, the One who sees the tears every month, and the One who listens alongside us when we hear the devastating doctor reports: "There is no hope for you to conceive," or "I hear no heartbeat."

Yes, He knows.

Whenever the harsh diagnosis and the disappointments arise, I've learned to lean into my partner Jesus and let His arms embrace me. I pour out my heart in prayer and He whispers sweet comfort into my ears. "It's alright, my child, follow my lead." As the longing for a child leaves me parched and dry, seeking Him through the Bible becomes living water to my soul and is consistent strength for me emotionally and physically.

The music strikes up again. He extends His hand toward me. I grasp it. He leads, I follow, and we move together as one on this infertility journey.

This is my desire and prayer for you.

As you learn to dance upon barren land, I pray the spiritual nourishment in this book will make the steps less cumbersome and ease you into the finale, the fertile field – parenthood.

As you pray each specific prayer, may your heavy heart find grace and may each prayer draw you into the dance, a relationship with Him. May the Scripture reflections bring comfort to your weary soul and physical healing to your lacking body.

While you wait, allow the seeds of character to develop within you. May the seeds of gifts and talents He has placed within you grow with purpose and blossom into hope, love, and encouragement for others.

Most of all, may the hurt and grief suffered through infertility and the sorrow from loss be replaced with joy, peace, and healing found through Jesus Christ. (Yes, it is possible. I am living proof.) And may you learn to *Dance Upon Barren Land*.

Blessed are you among women, and
blessed is the fruit of your womb!

Luke 1:42

Chapter 1
What is Prayer?

Barren land is a sparse, dark landscape of rocks, boulders, and at times massive cracks. The rocks and boulders, which cause us to stumble, are the repeated negative pregnancy tests, and the gritty sand is one of the many emotions such as jealousy, anger, or shame. Each month we hope and pray this is will be the month only to experience disappointment again, our hopes like shifting sand beneath our feet. Then after a miscarriage, stillbirth, or early infant loss, we face a massive crack of grief. We are unable to escape the darkness.

How does prayer fit into the vast and varied landscape of infertility?

As we call out to God in prayer, we are strengthened enough to kick the rocks of negativity out of the way and to pass through with ease and confidence. When we sink in the sand of disappointment, our petitions make our feet stable as we ask Him to come alongside and be our support. When our hearts are broken from the loss of life in our wombs and when we have sunk into the crevice of grief, when all we can muster is a faint cry, He still sees and hears.

So how do we navigate through the barren land with prayer?

There are four essential elements to each prayer:

- Praise
- Thanksgiving
- Praying the Word of God, the Bible
- Asking in Jesus' name

Praise and thanksgiving in prayer express our heart's adoration and love for Him.

> Enter His gates with thanksgiving and his courts with praise; give thanks to him and praise his name (Psalm 100:4).

The Bible explains itself in Hebrews 4:12:

> God's Word is living and powerful (NLT).

When we pray His Word, we are praying His perfect, divine will. What He did for infertile or barren women in the Bible so long ago—Sarah, Rebekah, Hannah, Manoah's wife, and Elizabeth—He can do for us.

> Jesus Christ is the same yesterday and today and forever (Hebrews 13:8).

God does not show favoritism (Acts 10:34).

The Lord Jesus Christ invites us to ask. Asking is for our benefit. We are told to ask, seek, and knock.

> Ask and it will be given to you; seek and you will find; knock and the door will be opened to you. For everyone who asks receives; those who seek find; and to those who knock, the door will be opened. Which of you, if your son asks for bread, will give him a stone? Or if he asks for a fish, will give him a snake? If you, then, though you are evil, know how to give good gifts to your children, how much more will your Father in heaven give good gifts to those who ask him! (Matthew 7:7-11).

When we ask in Jesus' name, we glorify Him and He fills us with joy.

> This is the confidence we have in approaching God: that if we ask anything according to his will, he hears us. And if we know that he hears us—whatever we ask—we know that we have what we have asked for (1 John 5:14-15).

21

The Bible and prayer are like nourishment for the soul and spirit. Prayer and Bible reading are like living water, which gives continual strength for the journey and increases faith to believe God for the desire of your heart: children.

Chapter 2
Why Pray these Prayers?

So, why should we pray these prayers?

Infertility throws hard punches. We can be wounded emotionally. Not only do the wounds interfere with our relationships, at times the medicines we are on for fertility treatments can either mask what we feel or heighten our emotions to a whole new level.

There are several reasons to pray:

- Peace
- Balance in relationships
- Deeper relationship with God

The first reason to pray is for peace of mind for us and in our relationships with others. In order to obtain peace that transcends all comprehension, the Bible encourages us to pray.

> Do not be anxious about anything, but in every situation, by prayer and petition, with thanksgiving, present your requests to God. And

the peace of God, which transcends all understanding, will guard your hearts and your minds in Christ Jesus (Philippians 4:6-7).

Praying to God is to posture ourselves in an act of surrender. You surrender to God by surrendering your heart. You can release your thoughts by telling Him of your worries, you can place your heightened emotions before Him by relating your painful experiences, and you can petition your desires to Him. However, the key to surrender is not giving up on life or the desire to become a parent but instead giving up anguish to the One who is able, Jesus Christ.

Oswald Chambers wrote, "It's not cowardly to pray when we are at our wit's end. It is the only way to get in touch with reality."[1]

Jesus instructed us to ask. He said, "Ask and it will be given to you; seek and you will find; knock and the door will be opened to you" (Matthew 7:7).

We should ask specifically and keep on asking. We find the perfect example in Hannah, once an infertile woman who became mother to Samuel, a prophet. Her story is found in the first chapter of 1 Samuel in the Old Testament. For years she desired a child. Each year the family went to the temple to worship. When Hannah prayed, she asked God to take note of her affliction. She was "in deep anguish, crying bitterly as she prayed to the Lord" (1 Samuel 1:10 NLT).

As she was praying, Eli, the priest, noticed her lips were moving yet she wasn't making a sound. He thought she was drunk and confronted her. She replied to him, "Oh no, sir! I'm not drunk! But I am very sad, and I was pouring my heart out to the Lord" (1 Samuel 1:15 NLT).

As Hannah poured out her heart before the Lord, she petitioned Him for the desire of her heart. God heard Hannah's prayer.

> Then they arose early in the morning and worshiped before the LORD, and returned again to their house in Ramah. And Elkanah had relations with Hannah his wife, and the Lord remembered her. It came about in due time, after Hannah had conceived, that she gave birth to a son; and she named him Samuel, saying, "Because I have asked him of the Lord." (1 Samuel 1:19-20 NASB).

> After the birth of a child, it was customary to return to the temple and dedicate your child to the Lord. At the time of Samuel's dedication, Hannah stood before Eli the priest and said, "As surely as you live, I am the woman who stood here

beside you praying to the Lord. I prayed for this child, and the Lord has granted me what I asked of him" (1 Samuel 1:26-27).

Author Beth Forbus suggests we look at this scene as if we were watching and replaying a video.

> I'd ask you to back the video up to 1 Samuel 1:27 when Hannah held her precious baby boy in her arms and looked at the priest Eli and said, "For this child I prayed, and the Lord has granted what I asked of Him ..." And then I'd ask you to replay and watch it again. And again. "For this child I prayed ..." Back it up and play, "For this child I prayed ..." Turn the volume up! "For this child I prayed ..." I can't help but believe if we could hear Hannah's voice when she said these words, we might just hear her passionate emphasis on the word "this." "For *THIS* child I prayed ..."[2]

In prayer, it's okay to keep asking for the desires of our hearts, even as we ask for peace in the pain of infertility. Our interactive communication with God fosters intimacy and trust in Him. Prayer lightens our heavy heart and helps to keep peace on this crazy journey.

Chapter 3
The Most Important Prayer
The Prayer of Salvation

The road of infertility is not an easy one to travel. Along the journey, you often feel alone and become weary, but there is Someone who desires to be your companion. He is the One who loves you, the One who can carry you through life, and the One who can help you reach your final destination: parenthood.

His name is Jesus Christ, God's one and only Son.

He is the lead partner in dancing upon barren land throughout infertility's song. The *Prayers* and *Scripture Reflections* in this book will help you, but the journey will be easier if you know Jesus Christ as your Lord and Savior. If you have not invited this companion into your life, it is simple; you can ask Him right now. Read the scriptures below, believe God gave His one and only Son for you, and then recite the prayer. Not only will you have His loving compassion and help along the fertility journey, but you are also guaranteed salvation, eternal life in heaven.

For God so loved the world that he gave his one and only Son, that whoever believes in him shall not perish but have eternal life (John 3:16).

Jesus answered, "I am the way and the truth and the life. No one comes to the Father except through me" (John 14:6).

If you confess with your mouth that Jesus is Lord and believe in your heart that God raised him from the dead, you will be saved. For it is by believing in your heart that you are made right with God, and it is by confessing with your mouth that you are saved (Romans 10:9-10).

To receive Christ as your Lord and Savior, believe and recite this prayer:

Dear Lord Jesus, I am a sinner and need Your forgiveness. I ask that you will come into my heart, to be my Lord and Savior. I trust You with my life. Thank You for the forgiveness of my sins and eternal life. I ask this in Your name, Amen.

Chapter 4
Prayers & Scripture Reflections for Infertility

Infertility and the longing for a child leave us parched; we need water for our dry and thirsting souls. Yet the only things to bubble up to the surface at unexpected and sometimes inconvenient times are our emotions. Situations sometimes ambush us and the pain is intense. When experiencing one of these situations or emotions, take the time to pray and read the Bible, then reflect and meditate on His Word. Use this book and these prayers to help you face down negative emotions.

- Pray the prayers.
- Read the supporting scriptures.
- Reflect on the words and promises; meditate.

The word "meditate" means "to engage in mental exercise for the purpose of reaching a heightened level of spiritual awareness; to reflect and ponder over."[3] Reflecting on God's Word will be like first aid, or living water, as you travel through the emotional spectrum of infertility. Reflection and meditation increase your faith to believe God to be your help and support. His Word can heal you from the grief of infertility and build hope to believe for the desires of your heart.

The prayer topics listed in this book come from many women and their experiences with infertility. Each topic is supported by Scripture and written for you to pray aloud or silently. You can recite the prayer as it is written or read the verses corresponding with the topic in the *Scripture Reflection* and make a personal prayer of your own.

Prayer is not a magical formula to get what you want; it's simply a way of communicating with God.

AGE
Prayer

Heavenly Father, my biological clock is ticking, as if You didn't know. As each month passes, I feel as if I am racing against that clock. Even the doctors speak of the impossibility of bearing children at my age. However, I praise You for Your Word, which has not left me hopeless. In Your Word I witness the creative power through the lives of Sarah and Elizabeth who bore children in their old age. Jesus, You say You are the same yesterday, today, and forever. If You did it for them so many years ago, today, I believe You can do it for me. As You say, nothing is impossible for You. Thank You for working possibility into my life.

In Jesus' name, amen.

Scripture Reflection

Abraham fell facedown; he laughed and said to himself, "Will a son be born to a man a hundred years old? Will Sarah bear a child at the age of ninety?"

Genesis 17:17

The righteous will flourish like a palm tree, they will grow like a cedar of Lebanon; planted in the house of the Lord, they will flourish in the courts of our God. They will still bear fruit in old age, they will stay fresh and green, proclaiming, "The Lord is upright; he is my Rock, and there is no wickedness in him."
Psalm 92:12-15

But they had no children, because Elizabeth was barren; and they were both well along in years.... After this, his wife became pregnant and for five months remained in seclusion.
Luke 1:7, 24

For nothing is impossible with God.
Luke 1:37

Jesus Christ is the same yesterday, today and forever.
Hebrews 13:8

ANGER
Prayer

Lord Jesus, I feel so angry and frustrated about my fertility challenges. I ask for Your divine love to flow through me, for Your love is patient and kind and not easily angered. Help me to be slow in my speech and slow in anger when it comes to dealing with my family members, friends, or doctor. Help me not to be angry with You, God, for all I am going through and for what I don't understand. Most of all, keep me from sinning against You or anyone else in my anger. Thank You, Father, for the release from anger within my heart.

In Jesus' name, amen.

Scripture Reflection

A hot tempered man stirs up strife, but the slow to anger calms a dispute.
Proverbs 15:18 NASB

Love is patient, love is kind. It does not envy, it does not boast, it is not proud. It is not rude, it is not self-seeking, it is not easily angered, it keeps no record of wrongs. Love does not delight in evil but rejoices with the truth. It always protects, always trusts, always hopes, always perseveres.

1 Corinthians 13:4-7

In your anger do not sin: Do not let the sun go down while you are still angry.

Ephesians 4:26

My dear brothers, take note of this: Everyone should be quick to listen, slow to speak and slow to become angry, for man's anger does not bring about the righteous life that God desires.

James 1:19-20

ANXIOUS
Prayer

Prince of Peace, a feeling of anxiousness has come over me. At times, my mind is racing and my heart beats fast. Father, help me to do as You say in Your Word. In prayer and petition and with a thankful heart, I let my requests be made known to You. As I lay my requests at Your feet, I exchange my anxious thoughts for a mind of peace, perfect peace as You have promised, when my mind is stayed upon You. I praise You for the peace that passes all understanding.
In Jesus' name, amen.

Scripture Reflection

You will guard him and keep him in perfect and constant peace whose mind [both its inclination and its character] is stayed on You, because he commits himself to You, leans on You, and hopes confidently in You.
Isaiah 26:3 AMP

Do not be anxious about anything, but in everything, by prayer and petition, with thanksgiving, present your requests to God. And the peace that passes all understanding will guard your heart and mind through Christ Jesus. Philippians 4:6-7

ABORTION

Sometimes a woman may feel infertility is a result of punishment for something in her past, such as abortion, but nothing could be further from the truth.

Prayer

Father God, You are the Giver of life. You say, "For you created my inmost being; you knit me together in my mother's womb." My heart is broken and I am emotionally numb. I made the choice to have an abortion and to remove life from me. I was overwhelmed, and made the choice out of misunderstanding and convenience. There was so much pressure on me. I am grieved by what I did. I am more than sorry. I ask for your forgiveness. You promised to "forgive all my sins...and crown me with loving kindness and compassion." I receive your forgiveness and I thank you for your love for me. My action condemns and haunts me. I cannot escape my thoughts. I thank You, "there is no condemnation for those who are in Christ Jesus." I ask for freedom from condemning, shameful thoughts and healing for my emotional wounds. You said, "Choose life that you and your children may live." From this moment forward, "I choose life." and I ask for another gift of a child to one day be "as a happy mother of children."

In Jesus' name, amen.

Scripture Reflection

For you created my inmost being; you knit me together in my mother's womb.
Psalm 139:13

Who forgives all your sins and heals all your diseases, who redeems your life from the pit and crowns you with love and compassion.
Psalm 103:3-4

Therefore, there is now no condemnation for those who are in Christ Jesus.
Romans 8:1

This day I call heaven and earth as witnesses against you that I have set before you life and death, blessing and curses. Now choose life, so that you and your children may live.
Deuteronomy 30:19

Behold, children are a gift of the LORD, The fruit of the womb is a reward.
Psalm 127:3

He settles the barren woman in her home as a happy mother of children.
Psalm 113:9

Instead of your shame you will receive a double portion, and instead of disgrace you will rejoice in your inheritance. And so you will inherit a double portion in your land, and everlasting joy will be yours.
Isaiah 61:7

ADOPTION
Prayer

Abba Father, as we have sought You through this infertility battle, You have placed the desire in us to grow our family through adoption. Thank You for setting apart our children before they were born and placing them with us. We ask You to order our steps and surround us with favor as a shield during this adoption process. Father, give us wisdom and discernment as we meet with officials—the adoption agency, social workers, court-appointed officials—and complete the necessary home study and paperwork. We ask You to release us from unnecessary guilt the enemy would try to place upon us for choosing adoption, knowing we've been trusting You from the start with the desire for a family. We thank You, for we know You'll work all these things for our good, the good of the birth parents, and our children yet to come. In Jesus' name, amen.

Scripture Reflection

Before I formed you in the womb I knew you, before you were born I set you apart ...
Jeremiah 1:5

Surely, Lord, you bless the righteous; you surround them with your favor as with a shield.
Psalm 5:12

God sets the lonely in families.
Psalm 68:6

Do justice to the weak [poor] and fatherless; maintain the rights of the afflicted and needy.
Psalm 82:3 AMP

But seek ye first the kingdom of God, and his righteousness; and all these things shall be added unto you.
Matthew 6:33 KJV

Therefore, there is now no condemnation for those who are in Christ Jesus.
Romans 8:1

And we know that in all things God works for the good of those who love him, who have been called according to his purpose.
Romans 8:28

If any of you lacks wisdom, you should ask God, who gives generously to all without finding fault, and it will be given to you.
James 1:5

41

BABY-RELATED HOLIDAYS
(Baby-Showers/Dedications/Christenings
Mother's Day/Father's Day)
Prayer

Almighty God, it seems as if every time I turn around I am faced with a celebration involving a baby. In my heart, I don't want to be jealous, angry, or envious, but it is hard to face these days. You said in Your Word You would go before me and be with me. You have not forsaken me and You are with me at each celebration. I ask for my focus to be outward toward others rather than inward toward myself. I pray for blessings on the new life being welcomed into this world with gifts and words and blessings. I thank You for all the mothers and fathers who are being celebrated on these special days. As I feel compelled to attend the event out of duty, I ask You to dissolve away my heaviness and strengthen me according to Your Word. Most of all, I thank You in advance for the day I will celebrate the blessing of my own children.

In Jesus' name, amen.

Scripture Reflection

The Lord himself goes before you and will be with you; he will never leave you nor forsake you. Do not be afraid; do not be discouraged.
Deuteronomy 31:8

Anger is cruel, and wrath is like a flood, but jealousy is even more dangerous.
Proverbs 27:4 NLT

My life dissolves and weeps itself away for heaviness; raise me up and strengthen me according to [the promises of] Your word.
Psalm 119:28 AMP

Rejoice with those who rejoice.
Romans 12:15

Give thanks in all circumstances, for this is God's will for you in Christ Jesus.
1 Thessalonians 5:18

BROKEN HEART
Prayer

Compassionate Father, my heart is crushed from this infertility battle. My emotions are frazzled. Lord, You said in Your Word You are close to the brokenhearted and save those who are crushed in spirit. I feel as if my reproductive system and my heart have failed. I cry out to You and I thank You; You are the strength of my heart and my portion. Come, Lord Jesus, be my refuge and bind up and heal my broken heart.

In Jesus' name, amen.

Scripture Reflection

The Lord is close to the brokenhearted and saves those who are crushed in spirit.
Psalm 34:18

My flesh and my heart may fail, but God is the strength of my heart and my portion forever.
Psalm 73:26

I cry to you, O Lord; I say, "You are my refuge, my portion in the land of the living."
Psalm 142:5

44

He heals the brokenhearted and binds up their wounds.
Psalm 147:3

CONCEPTION
Prayer

Creator God, thank You that I am fearfully and wonderfully made by You. I desire faith like Abraham, believing that You exist and that You reward those who diligently seek You. You said I would find You, God, when I seek You with all of my heart. Father, I choose to seek You first along this fertility journey. I praise You as You said in the Bible You would bless the fruit of my womb, and said to the Israelites that the number of their days You would fulfill, and that none will be barren among your people. I thank You that You are the same yesterday, today, and forever and Your promises are "Yes" and "Amen." What You did for the Israelites, I believe You can do for me. I thank You infertility and sterility have been nailed to the cross of Calvary through the sacrifice of Your dear Son, Jesus Christ. I thank You now for giving me faith and hope to believe for a miracle. In Jesus' name, amen.

Scripture Reflection

If you pay attention to these laws and are careful to follow them, then the Lord your God will keep

his covenant of love with you, as he swore to your forefathers. He will love you and bless you and increase your numbers. He will bless the fruit of your womb.
Deuteronomy 7:12-13

He settles the barren woman in her home as a happy mother of children.
Psalm 113:9

I praise you because I am fearfully and wonderfully made; your works are beautiful, I know that full well.
Psalm 139:14

But seek first his kingdom and his righteousness, and all these things will be given to you as well.
Matthew 6:33

Even Elizabeth your relative is going to have a child in her old age, and she who was said to be barren is in her sixth month. For nothing shall be impossible with God.
Luke 1:36-37

For no matter how many promises God has made, they are "Yes" in Christ. So through him the "Amen" is spoken by us to the glory of God.
2 Corinthians 1:20

Now faith is being sure of what we hope for and certain of what we do not see.
Hebrews 11:1

Jesus Christ is the same yesterday and today and forever.
Hebrews 13:8

And without faith it is impossible to please God, because anyone who comes to him must believe that he exists and that he rewards those who earnestly seek him.
Hebrews 11:6

By faith Abraham, even though he was past age—and Sarah herself was barren—was enabled to become a father because he considered him faithful who had made the promise.
Hebrews 11:11

DECISIONS
Prayer

Sovereign Lord, I thank You that You have the perfect plan to bring about a family in my life. Father, I am faced with the decision to _____. I ask You to instruct me and teach me in the way I should go. As Your eye is upon me, counsel me along this fertility journey. Since You consecrate life before it is born, I pray for Your help in my decisions to uphold the sanctity of life. Thank You, Father, for leading me in peace.

In Jesus' name, amen.

Scripture Reflection

Before I formed you in the womb I knew you, before you were born I set you apart; I appointed you as a prophet to the nations.
Jeremiah 1:5

I will instruct you and teach you in the way you should go; I will counsel you and watch over you.
Psalm 32:8

DIFFICULT RELATIONSHIPS
Prayer

Sovereign Lord, this fertility journey is not easy on my relationship with others. Help me to be silent or to watch what I say. Let no unwholesome word come out of my mouth. Help me to speak with wisdom, kindness, and compassion. For my husband/wife, the one You gave as my partner in life, I ask for Your help to respect his or her desires for a family. Help me with my mother, father, and other family members, to love and honor each one, even though none seems to understand our decisions on this fertility journey. I pray for my feelings about my friends. Help me not to take an offense at the silence about my fertility issues or to be hurt by anything that is said or done. I praise You that I am free to love those around me because of Your great love for me.

In Jesus' name, amen.

Scripture Reflection

Honor your father and your mother, so that you may live long in the land the Lord your God is giving you.

Exodus 20:12

A friend loves at all times, and a brother is born for adversity.
Proverbs 17:17

She speaks with wisdom, and faithful instruction is on her tongue.
Proverbs 31:26

So in everything, do to others what you would have them do to you, for this sums up the Law and the Prophets.
Matthew 7:12

And when you stand praying, if you hold anything against anyone, forgive him, so that your Father in heaven may forgive you your sins.
Mark 11:25

Love is patient, love is kind. It does not envy, it does not boast, it is not proud. It is not rude, it is not self-seeking, it is not easily angered, it keeps no record of wrongs. Love does not delight in evil but rejoices with the truth. It always protects, always trusts, always hopes, always perseveres.
1 Corinthians 13:4-7

Do not let any unwholesome talk come out of your mouths, but only what is helpful for building others up according to their needs, that it may benefit those who listen. And do not grieve the Holy Spirit of God with whom you were sealed for the day of redemption. Get rid of all bitterness, rage and anger, brawling and slander, along with every form of malice. Be kind and compassionate to one another, forgiving each other, just as in Christ God forgave you.
Ephesians 4:29-32

However, each one of you also must love his wife as he loves himself, and the wife must respect her husband.
Ephesians 5:33

DIRECTION
Prayer

Everlasting God, I ask that You will fulfill Your purpose for my life, my desire for children. Help me not to lean upon my own understanding or to rationalize the thoughts in my head. When there is a fork in the road and I don't know which path to take, I ask You to direct a straight path on this fertility journey. Teach me to know when to move forward or to stop or to rest along the way. As I put my trust in You, I thank and praise You that You are perfecting every little detail that concerns me.

In Jesus' name, amen.

Scripture Reflection

The Lord will fulfill his purpose for me; your love, O Lord, endures forever — do not abandon the works of your hands.
Psalm 138:8

Trust in the Lord with all your heart and lean not on your own understanding; in all your ways acknowledge him, and he will make your paths straight.
Proverbs 3:5-6

DISAPPOINTMENT
Prayer

Heavenly Father, it seems as if every month brings disappointment because I pray for a child and nothing happens. I don't understand why I have to suffer like this. In Your Word You said I am to rejoice in my sufferings because it gives me perseverance for the journey ahead, and perseverance brings about better character in me, and character brings hope. I praise You for Your great love, which has been shed in my heart by Your Holy Spirit. You give me hope that does not disappoint as I continue to believe in You. Thank You.

In Jesus' name, amen.

Scripture Reflection

Not only so, but we also rejoice in our sufferings, because we know that suffering produces perseverance; perseverance, character; and character, hope. And hope does not disappoint us, because God has poured out his love into our hearts by the Holy Spirit, whom he has given us.

Romans 5:3-5

For this is contained in Scripture: "Behold, I lay in Zion a choice stone, a precious corner stone, and he who believes in him will not be disappointed."

1 Peter 2:6 NASB

FACING ANOTHER WHO IS PREGNANT
Prayer

Faithful God, everywhere I turn, I see a pregnant belly. The very thing I desire is all around me. Help my eyes and my heart to turn upward toward You instead of outward upon others. When I see another who is pregnant, or hear of an unplanned pregnancy, help me not to become angry or resentful. Remind me how You've known this child even before You formed him in his mother's womb. This baby is part of Your ultimate, perfect plan. I ask You to bless these pregnancies and children yet to be born. You are no respecter of persons and what You've done for them You are faithful to do for me.
In Jesus' name, amen.

Scripture Reflection

After Job had prayed for his friends, the Lord made him prosperous again and gave him twice as much as he had before.
Job 42:10

Do not be eager in your heart to be angry, for anger resides in the bosom of fools.
Ecclesiastes 7:9 NASB

While I was fainting away, I remembered the Lord, and my prayer came to You, into Your holy temple.
Jonah 2:7 NASB

I most certainly understand now that God is not one to show partiality ....
Acts 10:34 NASB

By faith even Sarah herself received ability to conceive, even beyond the proper time of life, since she considered Him faithful who had promised.
Hebrews 11:11 NASB

FEAR
Prayer

Heavenly Father, I seek You who promised to answer me and deliver me from all my fears. I praise You because You are with me. I have no need to feel discouraged or afraid for my future or any fertility issues that may lie ahead. Thank You that You are my strength and my help. Bring peace to my troubled heart as You uphold me with Your righteous right hand. Father, help me overcome the fear of being forgotten and the fear of rejection from my family and friends. Help me not to fear becoming pregnant or pregnancy itself and help me overcome the fear of seeing a doctor and the tests, procedures, or studies involved. Remove my fear about not being chosen as an adoptive parent. Most of all, I ask for Your continual perfect love over me which casts out all fear, and I thank You for it.

In Jesus' name, amen.

Scripture Reflection

I sought the Lord, and he answered me; he delivered me from all my fears.
Psalm 34:4

So do not fear, for I am with you; do not be dismayed, for I am your God. I will strengthen you and help you; I will uphold you with my righteous right hand.
Isaiah 41:10

Peace I leave you; My peace I give to you; not as the world gives do I give to you. Do not let your heart be troubled, nor let it be fearful.
John 14:27 (NASB)

There is no fear in love. But perfect love drives out fear, because fear has to do with punishment. The one who fears is not made perfect in love.
1 John 4:18

FINANCES
Prayer

Mighty One, You know the path we are to take even before the first step. You see how our fertility challenges have brought us to the place of making major financial decisions. Father, give us wisdom regarding our finances as we seek Your direction for our future children. We believe Your Word and praise You that You will supply all of our needs according to Your riches in glory through Christ Jesus. Father, we will be obedient to Your Word to honor You with our wealth and with our tithe and offerings. Thank You for Your abundance in our finances.
In Jesus' name, amen.

Scripture Reflection

Honor the Lord with your wealth, with the first fruits of all your crops; then your barns will be filled to overflowing, and your vats will brim over with new wine.
Proverbs 3:9-10

"Will a man rob God? Yet you rob me. "But you ask, 'How do we rob you?' "In tithes and offerings. You are under a curse – the whole nation of you – because you are robbing me. Bring the whole tithe into the storehouse that

there may be food in my house. Test me in this," says the Lord Almighty, "and see if I will not throw open the floodgates of heaven and pour out so much blessing that you will not have room enough for it."
Malachi 3:8-10

And my God will meet all your needs according to his glorious riches in Christ Jesus.
Philippians 4:19

FORGOTTEN
Prayer

Precious Savior, I praise You that You were pleased to make me Your own and have accepted me in the beloved family of God because of Your dear Son, Jesus Christ. Father, these fertility challenges have made me feel forsaken and forgotten. I feel as if no one sees or cares about my desire for children. However, today I will make the choice to believe Your Word, not to be led by my feelings. Your Word tells me I am not hidden from Your sight, You won't leave me as an orphan, and You know every detail of my life, even the number of hairs on my head. You declare me worth more than any sparrow. Thank You. I praise You that nothing can separate me from Your love, not now or forever.

In Jesus' name, amen.

Scripture Reflection

For the sake of his great name the Lord will not reject his people, because the Lord was pleased to make you his own.
1 Samuel 12:22

Can a mother forget the baby at her breast and have no compassion on the child she has borne? Though she may forget, I will not forget you.
Isaiah 49:15

Are not two sparrows sold for a penny? Yet not one of them will fall to the ground apart from the will of your Father. And even the very hairs of your head are all numbered. So do not be afraid; you are worth more than many sparrows.
Matthew 10:29-31

And surely I am with you always, to the very end of the age.
Matthew 28:20

I will not leave you as orphans: I will come to you.
John 14:18

Who shall separate us from the love of Christ? Shall trouble or hardship or persecution or famine or nakedness or danger or sword? As it is written: "For your sake, we face death all day long; we are considered as sheep to be slaughtered." No, in all these things we are more than conquerors through him who loved us. For I am convinced that neither death nor life, neither

neither angels nor demons, neither the present nor the future, nor any powers, neither height nor depth, nor anything else in all creation, will be able to separate us from the love of God that is in Christ Jesus our Lord.
Romans 8:35-39

To the praise of the glory of his grace, wherein he hath made us accepted in the beloved.
Ephesians 1:6 KJV

And there is no creature hidden from His sight, but all things are open and laid bare to the eyes of Him with whom we have to do.
Hebrews 4:13 NASB

FUTURE
Prayer

Shepherd of my soul, I praise You because You have created me and have a perfect plan for my life. I thank You for Your desire to prosper me, not to harm me, to give me hope and a future. You have started this good work in me and I ask that You will perfect it until the day of Christ Jesus. Even though I don't understand why I have to go through these fertility challenges, I believe that You are a God who's in control. I rest in the fact You hold my future and You are working all things together for my good. Thank You.

In Jesus' name, amen.

Scripture Reflection

"For I know the plans I have for you," declares the Lord, "plans to prosper you and not to harm you, plans to give you hope and a future."
Jeremiah 29:11

And we know that in all things God works for the good of those who love him, who have been called according to his purpose.
Romans 8:28

… being confident of this, that he who began a good work in you will carry it on to completion until the day of Christ Jesus.
Philippians 1:6

GRIEF
Prayer

God of compassion, I praise You that You are the God of all comfort, too. I ask You to remove this burden of grief from my heart, for I believe You care for me. Thank You that You sent Your Son, Jesus Christ, who was acquainted and can identify with my sorrow and grief. I ask You to turn this mourning into joy, and I praise You that joy will be my strength for the days ahead. Thank You.

In Jesus' name, amen.

Scripture Reflection

Do not grieve, for the joy of the Lord is your strength.
Nehemiah 8:10

Surely our griefs He Himself bore, And our sorrows He carried.
Isaiah 53:4 NASB

The Lord will guide you always; he will satisfy your needs in a sun-scorched land and will strengthen your frame. You will be like a well-watered garden, like a spring whose waters never fail.
Isaiah 58:11

Praise be to the God and Father of our Lord Jesus Christ, the Father of compassion and the God of all comfort, who comforts us in all our troubles, so that we can comfort those in any trouble with the comfort we ourselves have received from God.

2 Corinthians 1:3-4

HEALING
Prayer

God my Healer, I thank You that You sent Your Son, Jesus Christ, to die on the cross for me. Your Son dying was not in vain but proved great benefits for me: the forgiveness of all my sin, past, present, and future, and the healing of all my diseases. Thank you that none of my fertility issues and/or sterility issues with my spouse are difficult for You. You tell me in Your Word that by Your great power and outstretched arm that nothing is too hard for You. I praise You for Your healing virtue in my life.

In Jesus' name, amen.

Scripture Reflection

He said, "If you listen carefully to the voice of the Lord your God and do what is right in his eyes, if you pay attention to his commands and keep all his decrees, I will not bring on you any of the diseases I brought on the Egyptians, for I am the Lord, who heals you."

Exodus 15:26

Praise the Lord, O my soul; all my inmost being, praise his holy name. Praise the Lord, O my soul, and forget not all his benefits—who forgives all your sins and heals all your diseases, who redeems

your life from the pit and crowns you with love and compassion.
Psalm 103:1-4

But he was pierced for our transgressions, he was crushed for our iniquities; the punishment that brought us peace was upon him, and by his wounds we are healed.
Isaiah 53:5

Ah, Sovereign Lord, you have made the heavens and the earth by your great power and outstretched arm. Nothing is too hard for you.
Jeremiah 32:17

Therefore confess your sins to each other and pray for each other so that you may be healed. The prayer of a righteous man is powerful and effective.
James 5:16

JEALOUSY and ENVY
Prayer

Loving Father, Your Word tells me how to love. I know being envious and jealous is not part of Your divine love. Father, I am struggling with envy and jealousy as I see pregnant women and hear of the birth of a new baby. Help me not to deny Your goodness and Your perfect plan for others as You bless them with children. Teach me not to compare my life with others, to take every negative, envious, and jealous thought captive to the obedience of Christ. Replace jealousy with genuine joy and envy with sincere gratitude. I ask Your help to rejoice in the truth with others as I hear of a pregnancy or birth. Thank You for teaching me Your way to love. In Jesus' name, amen.

Scripture Reflection

Love is patient, love is kind. It does not envy, it does not boast, it is not proud. It is not rude, it is not self-seeking, it is not easily angered, it keeps no record of wrongs. Love does not delight in evil but rejoices with the truth. It always protects, always trusts, always hopes, always perseveres.

1 Corinthians 13:4-7

We demolish arguments and every pretension that sets itself up against the knowledge of God, and we take captive every thought to make it obedient to Christ.
2 Corinthians 10:5

We do not dare to classify or compare ourselves with some who commend themselves. When they measure themselves by themselves and compare themselves with themselves, they are not wise.
2 Corinthians 10:12

MALE STERILITY
Prayer

Heavenly Father, Your Word said You formed my inward parts. I am fearfully and wonderfully made in Your image. You made me male and you gave us the command to be fruitful, to multiply, and to fill the earth. I ask You to complete in me what is lacking. I ask for the health of my reproductive system to prosper. I thank You for the desire You put in my heart to be a father. By faith, I believe that nothing is impossible with You.

In Jesus' name, amen.

Scripture Reflection

God blessed them and said to them, "Be fruitful and increase in number; fill the earth and subdue it."
Genesis 1:28

I praise you because I am fearfully and wonderfully made; your works are wonderful, I know that full well.
Psalm 139:14

For nothing is impossible with God.
Luke 1:37

Beloved, I pray that in all respects you may prosper and be in good health, just as your soul prospers.
3 John 2:2 NASB

MISCARRIAGE, STILLBIRTH, INFANT LOSS
Prayer

Merciful Father, the loss is heartbreaking. I feel as if I am walking through the valley of the shadow of death and as if I died a little, too. But Your Word tells me to fear no evil, for You are with me. Father, You said You would never leave me nor forsake me. I ask for your presence now to bless and comfort my heart as I mourn over the loss of life in my womb. I praise You when You say that You will give a full life span. I'm asking for my next pregnancy to be full term and our child full of life. Father, as I pray your Word I am believing and trusting You over my future. Thank You.

In Jesus' name, amen.

Scripture Reflection

Worship the Lord your God, and his blessing will be on your food and water. I will take away sickness from among you, and none will miscarry or be barren in your land. I will give you a full life span.

Exodus 23:25-26

No one will be able to stand up against you all the days of your life. As I was with Moses, so I will be with you; I will never leave you nor forsake you.
Joshua 1:5

Even though I walk through the valley of the shadow of death, I will fear no evil, for you are with me; your rod and your staff, they comfort me.
Psalm 23:4

Blessed are those who mourn, for they will be comforted.
Matthew 5:4

SECONDARY INFERTILITY
Prayer

God of abundance, I'm thankful for the one child You have given me but am struggling with guilt for desiring another. Your Word said there is no guilt or condemnation for those who are in Christ Jesus, so I ask You to free me! Even though my heart is heavy, I rejoice in You that You have the proper time and procedure for every matter. Help me to know how to answer my firstborn when he or she says, "I want a little brother or sister." Most of all, I am grateful for the child You have given and the perfect plan to bring the desire of my heart: another child.

In Jesus' name, amen.

Scripture Reflection

Though the fig tree does not bud and there are no grapes on the vines, though the olive crop fails and the fields produce no food, though there are no sheep in the pen and cattle in the stalls, yet I will rejoice in the Lord, I will be joyful in God my Savior.

Habbakuk 3:17-18

For there is a proper time and procedure for every matter, though a man's misery weighs heavily upon him.
Ecclesiastes 8:6

"For I know the plans I have for you," declares the Lord, "plans to prosper you and not to harm you, plans to give you hope and a future."
Jeremiah 29:11

SHAME, GUILT, CONDEMNATION
Prayer

Father God, I thank You that You have given Your Son, Jesus Christ, to die on the cross for all my sins, past, present, and future. Father, I draw near to You with a sincere heart in confidence, believing I have been cleansed from a guilty conscience. My fertility challenges make me to feel as if I am wearing a cloak of shame, guilt, and condemnation, but I choose to put on Your royal robe of righteousness. As I place my trust in You, knowing that I am Your child, I praise You; I will never be condemned or put to shame.

In Jesus' name, amen.

Scripture Reflection

I delight greatly in the Lord; my soul rejoices in my God. For he has clothed me with garments of salvation and arrayed me in a robe of righteousness, as a bridegroom adorns his head like a priest, and as a bride adorns herself with her jewels.

Isaiah 61:10

To you, O Lord, I lift up my soul; in you I trust, O my God. Do not let me be put to shame, nor let my enemies triumph over me.

Psalm 25:1-2

Then I acknowledged my sin to you and did not cover up my iniquity. I said, "I will confess my transgressions to the Lord"—and you forgave the guilt of my sin.
Psalm 32:5

Therefore, there is now no condemnation for those who are in Christ Jesus, because through Christ Jesus the law of the Spirit of life set me free from the law of sin and death.
Romans 8:1-2

As the Scripture says, "Anyone who trusts in him will never be put to shame."
Romans 10:11

... let us draw near to God with a sincere heart in full assurance of faith, having our hearts sprinkled to cleanse us from a guilty conscience and having our bodies washed with pure water.
Hebrews 10:22

STOPPING FERTILITY TREATMENTS
Prayer

Heavenly Father, as a couple we feel we should discontinue fertility treatments due to or because of _____. We believe when we married, You placed the desire in our hearts to have a family. We purpose to seek and delight in You and thank You as You bring about the desires of our hearts. Stopping treatment is hard and feels like failure and feels as if there is no plan or next step in sight, but we ask You to fill us with confidence and complete trust in You. We believe You'll bless and order our steps completing what You began in us—the desire for children.

In Jesus name, amen.

Scripture Reflection

But blessed is the man who trusts in the Lord, whose confidence is in him.
Jeremiah 17:7

The steps of a good man are ordered by the Lord: and he delighteth in his way.
Psalm 37:23 KJV

Trust in the Lord with all your heart and lean not on your own understanding; in all your ways acknowledge him, and he will make your paths straight.
Proverbs 3:5-6

... being confident of this, that he who began a good work in you will carry it on to completion until the day of Christ Jesus.
Philippians 1:6

TEST RESULTS
Prayer

Prince of Peace, as I await these test results I choose to cast down every imagination—fear, anxiety, and worry—bringing them into the captivity of Christ. I thank You that I have no need to fear bad news because You strengthen me and give me hope as I trust steadfastly in You. Help me understand the technical terms. Help me ask clear questions. Help the doctors guide the future protocol. My desire, O Lord, is to follow You.

In Jesus' name, amen.

Scripture Reflection

Free me from the trap that is set for me, for you are my refuge.
Psalm 31:4

So do not fear, for I am with you; do not be dismayed, for I am your God. I will strengthen you and help you; I will uphold you with my righteous right hand.
Isaiah 41:10

We demolish arguments and every pretension that sets itself up against the knowledge of God, and we take captive every thought to make it obedient to Christ.

2 Corinthians 10:5

He will have no fear of bad news; his heart is steadfast, trusting in the Lord.

Psalm 112:7

WAITING
Prayer

Gracious Father, waiting is hard, especially when I see pregnant women and little children. As I wait on the desire of my heart, help me to delight myself in You, to be strong and of good courage, and to wait for Your perfect plan. I praise and thank You as I wait on You. Restore my strength so I can soar like an eagle. I choose to place my trust in You in waiting, believing for the answer. Refresh me along this fertility journey.

In Jesus name, amen.

Scripture Reflection

Delight yourself in the Lord and he will give you the desires of your heart.
Psalm 37:4

I will wait for you, O Lord; you will answer, O Lord my God.
Psalm 38:15

I wait for the Lord, my soul waits, and in his word I put my hope.
Psalm 130:5

...but those who hope in the Lord will renew their strength. They will soar on wings like eagles; they will run and not grow weary, they will walk and not be faint.

Isaiah 40:31

WHEN MY SPOUSE AND I DISAGREE
Prayer

Gracious God, my quest to have a child has brought conflict into my marriage. I feel as if my spouse and I are divided. Father, (as a wife) I ask for help to adapt myself and to respect my husband and his decisions; Father, (as a husband) I ask for help to love my wife like Christ, to be understanding and not harsh toward her. As a couple, help our communication to be full of grace and our actions toward one another to be loving and kind. As we seek You and Your perfect plan, may we be at peace with one another and walk in agreement. I thank You that our fertility journey will not separate us but bring unity in our marriage now and for our future.

In Jesus' name, amen.

Scripture Reflection

The Lord will fight for you; you need only to be still.

Exodus 14:14

Can two people walk together without agreeing on the direction?

Amos 3:3 NLT

If possible, so far as it depends on you, be at peace with all men.
Romans 12:18 NASB

However, each one of you also must love his wife as he loves himself, and the wife must respect her husband.
Ephesians 5:33

Wives, submit yourselves to your husbands, as is fitting in the Lord.
Colossians 3:18

Let your speech always be with grace, as though seasoned with salt, so that you will know how you should respond to each person.
Colossians 4:6 NASB

WHEN PEOPLE SAY INSENSITIVE THINGS
Prayer

Heavenly Father, why do people say unkind things? I've been hurt by their words and insensitivity. Help me not to be offended, angry, or bitter because of what is said. Instead, help me to forgive. Help me hold my tongue so I won't lash out. Strengthen me in love so when I encounter insensitive words again I will not repay insult with insult but with blessing. Help others hear themselves and help me hear You.
In Jesus' name, amen.

Scripture Reflection

Cease from anger and forsake wrath; Do not fret; it leads only to evildoing.
Psalm 37:8 NASB

Set a guard over my mouth, O Lord; keep watch over the door of my lips.
Psalm 141:3 NASB

Bless those who persecute you [who are cruel in their attitude toward you]; bless and do not curse them.
Romans 12:14 AMP

Love is patient, love is kind. It does not envy, it does not boast, it is not proud. It is not rude, it is not self-seeking, it is not easily angered, it keeps not record of wrongs.
1 Corinthians 13:4-5

Finally, be strong in the Lord and in his mighty power.
Ephesians 6:10

See to it that no one misses the grace of God and that no bitter root grows up to cause trouble and defile many.
Hebrews 12:15

Do not repay evil with evil or insult with insult, but with blessing, because to this you were called so that you may inherit a blessing.
1 Peter 3:9

WHOLENESS AND COMPLETENESS
Prayer

Almighty Father, when You made creation, man and woman, You looked upon them and said that it was very good. Father, my empty womb has caused me to feel bad, like less of a woman, incomplete (or less of a man, incomplete). Father in heaven, as Your Word says, through faith in You, help me to endure this fertility journey. I thank You I am complete in spirit, soul, and body, lacking in nothing.

In Jesus' name, amen.

Scripture Reflection

God saw all that he had made, and it was very good.
Genesis 1:31

... and you have been given fullness in Christ, who is the head over every power and authority.
Colossians 2:10

Perseverance must finish its work so that you may be mature and complete, not lacking anything.
James 1:4

Chapter 5
Living Life While You Wait
A Personal Note

Infertility's song continues and it seems as if the dance through the barren land will never end. The song repeats. We push the stop button incessantly, but to no avail. We press pause and the best we get is a change of tune to "While I'm Waiting."

In the previous chapters, we've learned how to navigate the land of infertility through prayer, and we've discovered how reading the Bible helps us survive the varied and vast landscape. But what do we do while we wait?

We learn to live life. Living is what I learned to do.

The key to living life is found in Scripture.

> Return our fortunes, Lord, as streams renew the desert. Those who plant in tears will harvest with shouts of joy. They weep as they go to plant their seed, but they sing as they return with the harvest (Psalm 126:4-6 NLT).

There are five distinguishable words in this verse:

- tears
- weep
- seed
- plant
- harvest

These fundamental words are vital to health and joy. Your tears and weeping are a prelude to living life to the fullest. The next step is the seed. Before sprouting, a seed goes through a period of dormancy. The seed "survives adverse climate conditions until circumstances are favorable for growth."[4] God has planted a seed of desire for children into your heart, but you face infertility. He has also placed many other seeds into your life, which you can develop while you wait:

- Seeds of character
- Seeds of giving
- Seeds of talent

In order for a seed to grow, it must be nurtured and watered. The tears we cry because of infertility moisten the seeds of character and giving and talent within us. Our weeping changes the hard, dry, barren landscape of our hearts to a soft, green fertile field. As we plant seeds in the act of giving to others, we receive an abundant harvest in unexpected ways. Infertility has a way of pushing us into a land we've never been before, but watering the seeds of talent within us will enable us to enjoy life while we wait.

Seeds of Character

Infertility is one of the most heart-wrenching, emotional roller coaster rides we can ride. The testing of jealousy, anger, and shame, to name a few, is at each downhill slope, turn, and twist. The ride is a process of dealing with the psychological reactions reaching to the core of who we really are.

One cold Christmas season our dear friends JoAnn and Milt came to our home. We planned to go out to dinner that evening. They had moved back to Houston from Atlanta, so we were looking forward to getting together again. As we sat in the living room surrounded by the glow of the twinkling lights and scent of the cedar Christmas tree, they announced the news, "We didn't expect it to happen quickly, but we're expecting."

Their announcement added to the joy and warmth of the season of Christmas; however, the atmosphere of my heart turned from warm to cold. We proceeded to dinner to one of our favorite Italian restaurants. The smell of garlic bread permeated the air, yet it didn't stir my appetite. Throughout the course of the meal, our conversation sounded to me like the teacher from the cartoon show *Charlie Brown*, as if I was in a glass bubble.

Later that evening, I happened to be home alone. I felt so angry and I'd had enough. I began to yell at God. Tears flowed. I held my Bible up to the heavens and yelled, "Why God? This is not fair! I have been married longer, and You put this desire in my heart first; why are You doing this to me?" My pitiful state resembled a volcano erupting, hot tears and bubbling snot streaming down my face. Yet ever so gently, I felt my Heavenly Father's loving kindness.

Are you going to stay angry and jealous, or are you going to pray for that unborn child?

Bull's-eye.

Ouch. God, that really hurts.

Then I repented of my selfish, jealous state.

Fast forward to a few years later. Now the child I prayed for while in my friend's womb is my li'l friend Matthew. Out of all the children I know, he is the one who comes running with open arms with a big, loud welcoming, "Hi,

Aunt Lesli." When he was a toddler, his mom and I would get together and somehow he'd make his way into my lap. Now that he's older, he always seems to make a way into my presence placing his arm around me. Upon leaving my friends' home, Matthew, whether in summertime in his socks or in winter barefooted, runs alongside my car as I drive off, laughing, and saying, "Goodbye, Aunt Lesli. Love you."

Infertility presents an opportune time to build our character. I would like to reflect upon these two scriptures. The word "seed" referenced here is in a different context. It's talking about the Word of God and you, the soil of your heart. He can change your heart from bitter to better.

> And the one on whom seed was sown on the good soil, this is the man who hears the word and understands it; who indeed bears fruit, and brings forth, some a hundredfold, some sixty, and some thirty (Matthew 13:23 NASB).

> Not only so, but we also glory in our sufferings, because we know that suffering produces perseverance; perseverance, character; and character, hope (Romans 5:3-4).

The seeds of character God has planted in me have not been easy.

So what about you? When a friend becomes pregnant, how will you respond? When your spouse disagrees with the expensive fertility treatment, how will you behave? When God doesn't answer your prayer as quickly as you'd like, will you allow anger or bitterness to set in?

When these things happen, whether we know it or not, or like it, God is working in us His good character, if we will allow Him to do so.

Recently, JoAnn and Milt had their fifth son. Yes, you read correctly; the number is five. One of the middle names of their last son is my maiden name. What an honor and a sense of validation for me. I could've stayed jealous and angry, but if I had, I wouldn't have my li'l friend Matthew, nor would I have this priceless, loyal friendship with JoAnn.

> Those who plant in tears will harvest with shouts of joy (Psalm 126:5 NLT).

Seeds of Giving

I love to garden. There is something about putting a seed into the ground, and returning in a few days to spot a tender green shoot. Yet before you see the beauty of the garden or taste its bountiful harvest, you must first deliberately plant a seed in the soil. A seed is tangible thing you plant or can give away. Sometimes I must give away what I desire most in order to reach out to others. Through my infertility, God has given me an opportunity to know Him in an unexpected way. Now I help others understand His love, even in the disappointment and grief of infertility.

As I dealt with my own pain, I had the desire to reach out to a local Christian infertility support group. I live in a large metropolitan area of four million plus people, so I assumed there would be at least one local group within the city of Houston, but none was listed. As I continued to search, I discovered the nearest Christian-based infertility support group was more than a five-hour drive away in Carrollton, Texas, near Dallas.

When I was a young girl, my wonderful mom taught me how to sew; and when I married, my precious mother-in-law taught me how to crochet trim around a blanket (which she learned from her ninety-year-old neighbor). The two skills combined helped me create a beautiful baby blanket.

I remembered reading about the history of women in Colonial America crafting "piecework." Women knitted and sewed garments for pay as a home business. So I had an idea. I composed an invitation to a "Peacework" party in my home. I asked my girlfriends to gather to learn a new skill with the goal of giving to the infertility support group.

I contacted the group leader in Carrollton; she was surprised by the thought and generosity, and eagerly welcomed my coming with the blanket gifts. She even asked if I would share my infertility story.

The gathering of women—mothers, daughters, aunts, friends—young and old alike, all fellowshipping and laughing, purposed with a common goal to make baby blankets was a desire accomplished. We had so much fun together. Our two-month project stretched into six months. Finally we finished and wrapped the baby blankets in ribbon, tagged with the sentiment "Stitched with Love, Hemmed by Prayer."

A hot August day arrived. The delivery day of the baby blankets. After church, my friend Jenn and I started out on our five-hour stretch along the Texas highway.

As I listened to the women's stories at the meeting, I was touched beyond tears. No words truly describe how much my heart moved with compassion. As I shared my journey, I told how I wanted to reach out to them in their pain. I handed each one a blanket. The women cried as they caressed the soft flannel and read the tag. It was a priceless moment for me.

As soon as we got in the car to return home, Jenn turned to me and said, "You need to start something like this."

I said, "Yeah, right. How would I do this, and where in the world would I do it?" But God was already at work. Within months, the wife of my pastor asked me to begin a Christian infertility support group through the women's ministry at the church. This was something I did not seek out on my own to do. I say this humbly, I strongly feel God used the seed I planted to bring a harvest to help others with infertility within the largest church in America, Lakewood Church, pastored by Joel Osteen.

HOPE ~ Hearts of Promise and Expectation for Women© Christian Infertility Support group is going strong after many years.

> They weep as they go to plant their seed, but they sing as they return with the harvest (Psalm 126:6 NLT).

Seeds of Talent

For me, after months of disappointment, no positive pregnancy news, and dealing with the horrid emotions of infertility, I came to realize I was in a box. I call it the "Me Want Baby Box!"

I felt as if I was sitting in this box; each of the walls was covered with photos, posters, and plaques about getting pregnant. Every direction I looked, I saw something dealing with a baby. Having a baby was all I could think about. Throughout the process of infertility, we can put ourselves in this box, trapped by our own desires. Phil Munsey said, "We tend to be so consumed with what we want, we lose sight of the fact of who we are."[5]

After our last fertility treatment, my husband and I sat in the doctor's office waiting for the pregnancy test results. The doctor sat across from us with a somber look and said, "I'm sorry, it is negative. With your age and your egg maturity, I feel there is no hope for you to conceive."

Her words pierced my soul. I felt like someone sucked the air out of the room and I was left lying on the floor. It was as if something died within my heart. That day was one of the most difficult days of my life. Thankfully, God's grace flooded me that evening. He healed me from my grief and sorrow and in those moments of pain; He brought joy and laughter (but that's a story for another book.).

The next morning I recall sitting at my breakfast table, praying emphatically aloud, "Devil, watch out. I have seeds to sow into women."

We went to dinner with some longtime friends, Carl and Jessica,[1] and they inquired about how the HOPE© support group was coming along.

I said, "I have this desire to reach out. I know there are more women out there hurting through infertility."

Carl said, "If you want to do that, we will help get you started."

Tears streamed down my face. My husband was talking to another guest at the table. He looked over and noticed me crying. Concerned, he asked, "Lesli, what's wrong?"

With the typical female response, I replied, "Oh, nothing." I was truly speechless because of the kind gesture of our friends.

That night their words validated a seed of talent in my heart, the call of God. The seed was dormant and lying as if lifeless in the soil of my life. The words of our friends brought the seed to life. Within months, I contacted their web designer who designs corporate websites, and the couple gave me $3,000 to start the online ministry.

---

[1] Names changed for privacy.

And my first baby was born: *Dancing Upon Barren Land ~ Spiritual Nourishment for the Infertility Road.* Now I minister to others around the world through the website and to local infertility support groups, which have formed in other churches, too. God has birthed a ministry and a joy in me beyond anything I could have dreamed.

Remember, a seed's stage of dormancy can "survive adverse conditions until circumstances are favorable for growth." I survived the adverse condition of the doctor's report, which pushed me into a favorable circumstance, the dinner with our friends, and essentially God's plan for my life. The seed of talent and ministry burst forth to produce beautiful fruit. Skills within me broke through to the surface – administrative aptitudes and creative gifts and relationship abilities. My dream of bearing a child still lies dormant, with the hope of sprouting soon, but a new dream of serving and giving hope to others blossomed.

Once I had horrible mixed feelings when a close friend became pregnant; I was so happy for her, yet jealous of her and so sad for me. On another day, a doctor's report crushed me to the core. In these times, the barrenness seemed to overwhelm me. Yet with kindness and gentleness, Jesus helped me overcome the pain, and each new day presents an opportunity to live life to the fullest.

Water and Nurture your Seeds

"Your heart is full of fertile seeds, waiting to sprout."[6]

God planted seeds in you, seeds to grow your character, seeds to help you become a giver, and seeds to use your talents. These seeds are glorious gifts from the Heavenly Father. Rejoice in Him. You are fearfully and wonderfully made by God. He created you to be beautiful and talented. He has given you life to live.

God is watching over us, and He has not forgotten about our dreams and desires. We can live each day by following some basic principles.

- Discover who you are in Christ by reading the Bible.
- Determine who you are as an individual. What are your passions?
- Take action: plant the first seed.
- Water and nurture the seeds of talent within you, and allow others to water your seeds of talent, too.

Yes, you have the God-given desire to be a mother or father, but what about you? You are more than your desire, just as you are more than any accomplishment.

So dance.

Infertility is a free ticket to no man's land—the desert, a travel destination we never planned for nor ever dreamed of visiting. We've been forced into a barren landscape. Yet infertility's land reaches the core of who we are in our emotions and reaches to the center of who God made us to be—complete and perfect in Him. The grief of infertility and the sorrow from loss leads us to live in pain or to live in abundant joy.

The choice is ours.

The rewards of living life to the fullest are found in the seeds along the path of infertility. There are seeds to develop the character of God, to give and plant into others, and to utilize the talents within us. Even though infertility's journey is difficult, the future is much more than we ever dreamed.

Yes, the tune "While You Wait" is still playing, and yes, the storm is hard, but the power and love of God are strong. My prayer is for God to turn your grief into joy and for you to see the prospects and potential in front of you. You've had broken expectations, but don't stop living. Seize every opportunity. Hold on to hope. Never lose your ability to see the world around you with wide-eyed curiosity.

The words from the book *Gift of the Red Bird* sum it up beautifully.

> But I am beginning to see that that journey was the only way to get my attention. It was the backdrop. If I were in a theater, that journey was the set design, the scenery, but now the real landscape is in front of me.[7]

As you've taken the lead partner's hand, the hand of Jesus Christ, I believe you're learning how to master the dance through the barren landscape of infertility. The massive cracks of grief are starting to close, and each step you take is surer. The seeds you've planted, watered by the living water of God's grace and love, have sprouted new life around you.

The music is beginning. The real landscape is in front of you.

Go ahead. Dance upon barren land.

When the Lord brought back His exiles to
Jerusalem, it was like a dream!

We were filled with laughter, and
we sang for joy.

And the other nations said,
"What amazing things the Lord has done
for them."

Yes, the Lord has done amazing things for
us! What joy!

Restore our fortunes, Lord,
as streams renew the desert.

Those who plant in tears
will harvest with shouts of joy.

They weep as they go to plant
their seed, but they sing as
they return with the harvest.

Psalm 126:1-6 NLT

Afterword

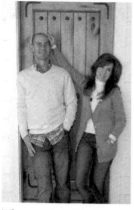

Some people dance to different tunes.

Every newly married couple encounters these different melodies after the sound of wedding bells fade. Larry and I discovered our differences not long after our honeymoon.

The goals of career and the purchase of a home delayed starting a family. Yet, for me, when the intense desire to have a child came, our differences showed up clearly. We didn't dance to the same tune. I wanted a song with a fast beat, to move forward in having children soon. Larry, on the other hand, wanted a slow dance; he wasn't in a hurry.

Larry and I were encouraged by others to write this *Afterword* together. Actually, it is me, Lesli, doing the writing. I'm the speller and writer of the family and Larry is the mathematician and financial expert. We work well that way. So we sat down together, to recount the years of our fertility journey, the trials we faced, and how each of us responded to one another. There were tears, then a chuckle, as we realized our first date was the first glimpse of our differences. We ordered opposites from the menu. Larry is Mr. Peanut Butter and Jelly and I'm Mrs. Gourmet.

Not only did our opposing views show up in family planning, but also, in how we expressed ourselves in our emotions and through our personalities. We are people of faith yet we expressed our beliefs and confidences in God in opposite ways too. The varying expressions didn't make either one of us right or wrong, but at times it led to hurt, misunderstanding, and confusion. Finally, over the years we've developed an understanding of one another. The journey to knowing and appreciating each other is a process; the journey takes time, and it takes the Word of God.

In anguished prayer, I begged God to allow me to become pregnant. My melancholy tendencies didn't help matters either. My intense longing pulled at Larry with almost a demand on him to pray for a child. When he wouldn't pray in the way I prescribed, I'd get upset. My pressure on him caused tension in our relationship. Larry is the type of guy who likes to have fun. He loves to inject humor everywhere he goes. For instance, one day as he gathered the mail he handed me a magazine with children on the cover, laughing as he said, "Here's some children for you." The shot of humor was not at the right time, nor was it the most thoughtful, but it's his personality. Larry is a very tender, loving man. He wanted to resolve my sadness, yet didn't know how to respond.

I realized I had to back off and not pressure him, to communicate without conditions taking Romans 15:18 to heart, "If possible, so far as it depends on you, be at peace with all men." Larry eventually saw through my façade and realized he needed to come alongside me with emotional support, as 1 Peter 3:7 states, "You husbands, likewise, live with your wives in an understanding way...." One day he said, "Lesli, I know you are on an emotional roller coaster, but a roller coaster has two seats and I'm sitting right next to you." How precious those comforting words.

Eventually, not pressuring, communicating without conditions, and directing my blubbering prayer requests to God led to a special gift. One day Larry said, "Lesli, if we are praying and believing for a child, we need to act on our faith and buy a crib." That crib is one of the most priceless gifts I've ever received from him.

I continued to pray with tears asking God to become a mother. On the other hand, Larry shouted to the rooftops, "Come on God, bring our Abigail." I would say, "Larry, it's not the right time of the month," and he'd respond, "Lesli, it doesn't matter what time of the month it is, God doesn't even need me." I've learned to appreciate his deep abiding faith – and his humor.

My desire for children is like an audition for a part in the dance. Backstage in the dimly lit room the dancer practices, prepares, and hopes to get the part. Yet I've never been called to dance the role of mother. Well, at least not yet anyway.

As we pondered the years of this hard journey, Larry said, "The enemy has put a wall in front of you. You've made the choice not to stay behind the wall, but to use the wall to leap over to the other side. Your compassion towards women facing the same situation as you is wonderful and amazing. You are doing so good."

Larry's words helped me fling open the heavy drapes of isolation, despair, and grief pushing aside the enemy's tactics. Like opening my heavy heart to the One, Jesus Christ and answering the call to the role of living life in "joy and peace in believing" (Romans 15:3) taking center stage and inviting others to dance with me.

Our desire for a child is not lost, neither is our faith in God. He can bring possibility to an impossible situation. There are days when I, Lesli, have an intense longing or sadness and days when Larry comes home choked up with tears, "I saw a little girl today; I wish I had one. She'd be my best bud. We could play together and I know she'd constantly say, 'Let's do it again Daddy!'"

We have children not born to us, but born of our heart and we love each one. We are known as Uncle Larry and Aunt Lesli to many children and young adults, apart from our own niece and nephew. We know God has positioned us as mentors with the privilege to speak into these lives. During the day it's the young adults who want to come over and 'play' (because Larry's still thinks he's 18), and it's in the midnight hour we'll receive a text and welcome with open arms a troubled soul.

We don't see our arms as empty, but our lives as full.

We've not been abandoned by God to wonder what He is up to, but are living this wonderful life freely given by Him. We have liberty to pursue our passions and His purposes are revealed to us. We love life and have come to understand each other in amazing ways.

Dancing faces you toward one another. No longer are you stepping on one another's toes or having to think about the next step or movement. There is intimacy and unity in whichever direction you turn. Ruth St. Denis said, "Dance communicates between body and soul to express what is too deep to find in words."[8] Our steps are in-sync now on this fertility journey and in our lives. Moving together as one, with empathy, love, and respect.

Now we are cheek to cheek, slow dancing to the same tune in this fast-paced world. The dance floor has plenty of room. Come on. Will you join us?

Acknowledgments

So many have helped me personally throughout the infertility journey and professionally in the creation of this book. More than just print on a page, my heartfelt love and appreciation extends to each one.

Karen Porter, my writing coach, editor, and mentor. Without your valuable knowledge in the Christian writing and speaking industry, your stability keeping me guided and grounded, as well as your belief in my talent, this book would not be possible. I'm indebted to you in the creation and production of this project. Thank you with all of my heart.

My husband, Larry, truly there is only one phrase: unconditional love. You are my consistent pillar of faith and pillow of comfort. The one who has been there in the depths of my despair, the one who believes in me, and whose joyous attitude towards life thrusts me forward each new day. I'm honored to share this life of love with you.

My family, the Coopers and the Westfalls. I've naturally inherited gifted traits from my family and those learned amongst my extended family members. A love and legacy of faith that knows no end. Truly I can say, "The lines have fallen to me in pleasant places; Indeed, my heritage is beautiful to me." Psalm 16:6. I love and appreciate each of you.

The Women of Hope, HOPE Christian Infertility Support Group at Lakewood Church. Through your shared experiences, I've received a broader view on how women deal with infertility and loss. I have learned how, our Savior Jesus Christ has been faithful to you on your journey. Truly, I have found my support in you and it is to you all I dedicate this book.

The Dancing Upon Barren Land Ministry Board, JoAnn Heath, April Jones, Larry Westfall, and Chris Whittington. Your financial support laid a foundation to begin this ministry and your faithful prayers enable me to reach those around the world who are struggling with infertility. Thank you for believing in me.

Lakewood Church pastoral leadership, Pastors' Joel and Victoria Osteen and Jackie Garner, Director of Women's Ministry, my appreciation, for extending the invitation and the opportunity to serve those who are grieving from infertility and infant loss throughout the greater Houston area. And to the extended Osteen family, Mrs. Dodie Osteen, Dr. Paul and Jennifer Osteen, and Lisa Osteen-Comes, thank you for your love and consistent support.

Allison Smythe and Wayne Leal of arsGraphica for their initial work for the website, with a special thanks to Allison for her beautiful designs for the book cover and logo. Thanks to Eric Forsythe of Forsythe Fotography for photo images and to OOA Productions, Harold Green and Larry Westfall for promotional videos.

My Peeps: Andrea Jones, Becki Guillory, JoAnn Heath, Renee Reagan, and Heather Volentine, "my five smooth stones," you all have been there before the beginning of this journey, during, and I know you'll be there until I reach the end of this barren road. Your friendship is my priceless treasure.

My Jesus, my Lord and Savior, my everything. It is in Him and by Him I have made it thus far. May He be honored and glorified in everything I say, write, and do. I love Him so.

Dancing Upon Barren Land Ministry

From childhood most women dream of having children of their own. Our culture has changed over the decades. Couples start families later in life. With the delayed parenting, infertility issues and woes increase and most women do not expect the delay or the pain.

It's estimated one out of six American couples experience infertility, and the numbers are higher worldwide. Infertility knows no boundaries when it comes to gender, race, culture, or belief in God. Essentially a childhood dream is shattered when the desire for children isn't fulfilled quickly or at all. In its wake, the crushed dream leaves an emotional strain on relationships, a financial drain for fertility treatments, and ultimately, a broken heart.

Where is a place of acceptance and inspiration for a confused mind and depleted heart?

Dancing Upon Barren Land – Spiritual Nourishment for the Infertility Road addresses those needs through a Christian online support ministry for all no matter if a person professes a belief in God or has never attended service in a church, synagogue, or temple. The non-profit organization offers inspiration and information through; resources for those suffering with infertility, prayers to nourish the barren soul, infertility etiquette to help friends and family understand, and a tool to help ministry leaders counsel those with infertility needs. The ministry's mission is to provide hope and healing from the grief of infertility and sorrow from loss through Jesus Christ.

Dancing Upon Barren Land connects women and couples locally through support groups and internationally through the website.

For more information:
www.DancingUponBarrenLand.com

Contact:
Dancing Upon Barren Land
P.O. Box 1054
Pearland, Texas 77588

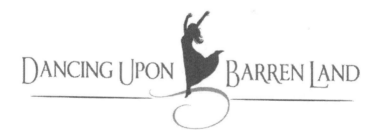

About Lesli Westfall

Lesli is no stranger to infertility. She has experienced all the range of emotions, the prodding of doctors, and the stinging disappointments. She's been left wandering on the barren road and has wondered what God is up to as she asked endless questions. Yet looking back on her journey, she realizes God turns disappointments into appointments with Him, the most significant being the call to offer hope and inspiration to the wounded heart of the barren soul.

While leading a Christian infertility support group in one of the largest churches in America, Lakewood Church pastored by Joel Osteen, a deep compassion formed.

Through her own experience and those shared from others, an online ministry was created *Dancing Upon Barren Land - Spiritual Nourishment for the Infertility Road.*

Now she ministers to women around the world through the website and leads local support groups, which have formed in other churches too.

Lesli enjoys life. She loves spending time with her husband, Larry, her man of faith and live-in comedian, and enjoys riding his entrepreneurial wave as well as her own, teaching cooking and etiquette to children. She loves spending time with her family and friends, and traveling, especially road trips. She adores eating dark chocolate.

Most of all, her passion is sharing God's love and teaching His Word to women, inspiring belief there's healing for the grief of infertility and sorrow from loss, and there is joy in the journey while we wait.

Other published works by Lesli,

"His Longing Lingers," *Moments of Grace*, 2008.

Want Lesli to speak at your next
conference, support group, or event?
You may contact Lesli through the website
www.DancingUponBarrenLand.com

Subscribe to Devotional Blog at:
www.DancingUponBarrenLand.com

Follow Dancing Upon Barren Land on:

 Dancing Upon Barren Land Ministry

 @DUBLhope

HOPE Support Groups

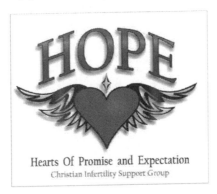

Hearts Of Promise and Expectation
Christian Infertility Support Group

Not having children can affect family relationships and friendships. Estrangement is felt in large crowds and in intimate gatherings of friends. For those suffering from infertility or loss, the once imagined identity of a mother is lost causing grief, a heartache not validated or acknowledged. For women, a connection to others is essential for their emotional well-being.

HOPE ~ Hearts of Promise and Expectation© is a group for women suffering from infertility, secondary infertility, miscarriage or failed adoption attempts. HOPE provides

- a safe place for shared feelings,
- strengthening in faith through the Bible,
- healing for the grief of infertility and sorrow from loss through prayer, and
- emotional and spiritual support through fellowship with others on a similar journey.

If you'd like to know more about a local support group, starting a group within your community or church, or to purchase resources, please contact us at www.DancingUponBarrenLand.com.

Discussions Topics for Support Groups

Chapter 1 - What is Prayer?

1. How has prayer fit into your journey through infertility?

2. There are four essential elements to prayer: praise, thanksgiving, praying the Word of God, the Bible, and asking in Jesus' name. How have these four elements been a part of your prayer life?

3. Which of the four elements of prayer have been missing in your prayer life?

 Action step: add the missing element to your prayer life.

Chapter 2 - Why Pray these Prayers?

1. Do you believe it is essential to pray? Why?

2. Listed in this chapter are several reasons to pray: peace, balance in relationships, and a deeper relationship

with God. Which of these three reasons do you struggle with the most?

3. In 1 Samuel 1:10, the Bible shows how Hannah was open to God and how she poured out her heart's desire for a child. Are you open to God when you pray?

 Action step: it's never too late to start praying. Start now.

Chapter 3 - The Most Important Prayer - The Prayer of Salvation

Note to Small Group Leader: Use this chapter as a guide to lead members of your small group into the prayer of salvation and a relationship with Jesus Christ.

Chapter 4 - Prayer and Scripture Reflection for Infertility

1. Describe the most painful emotion you have experienced through infertility?

2. From the Prayer Topics listed in the chapter, which three topics do you find yourself praying most frequently? Why?

3. Has prayer been helpful to you throughout infertility? Describe what prayer means to you.

 Action step: continue praying until there is peace within you and your relationship with others becomes balanced. Prayer will draw you closer to God.

Chapter 5 - Living Life While You Wait

1. Lesli describes the life cycle of a seed. A seed will "survive adverse climate conditions until circumstances are favorable for growth." Presently, what adverse condition of infertility are you facing?

2. Lesli mentions that there are many "seeds to plant,"— seeds of character, seeds of giving, and seeds of talent.

What seeds of character has God sown in you?

3. Are you planting seeds of giving? If so, describe.

4. List your seeds of talent. Or better yet, have a friend or family member list your seeds of talent. Describe how your seeds of talent are being used?

 Action step: start sowing seeds to others and water the seeds of talent within you.

Afterword

1. Describe the differing viewpoints you and your spouse have (or have had) during infertility.

2. Have these different viewpoints caused conflict? If so, explain.

3. Lesli wrote: "Her intense longing pulled at Larry with almost a demand on him to pray for a child." Has your intense longing for child placed demands upon your spouse? If so, how?

4. How are your *emotions* expressed through your personality type? How do they differ from your spouse?

5. How is your *faith* expressed through your personality type? How does it differ from your spouse?

6. As a couple, how have you resolved conflict?

 Action step: list some steps you and your spouse can take to "dance to the same tune." and come to conflict resolution.

Chapter 2

[1] Oswald Chambers, *If You will Ask*, Oswald Chambers Publication Assoc. 2nd Edition, (1989) 15.

[2] Beth Forbus, "Daily Double Portion," Sarah's Laughter Ministry, http://www.sarahs-laughter.com/daily-double-portions.html, 12/18/2012.

Chapter 4

[3] Merriam- Webster's Dictionary Online, "meditate" http://www.merriam-webster.com/dictionary/meditate.

Chapter 5

[4] Wikipedia, "seed" http://en.wikipedia.org/wiki/seed.

[5] Author's notes Phil Munsey, Lakewood Church, 2012.

[6] Moreihei Ushiba, http://www.brainyquote.com/quotes/authors/m/morihei_ueshiba_2.html, 12/18/12.

[7] Paula, D'Arcy, *Gift of the Red Bird,* The Crossroad Publishing Co., 1996, 53.

Afterword

[8] Ruth St. Denis, http://www.brainyquote.com/quotes/authors/r/ruth_st_denis.html, 12/18/2012.